Sugar Detox For Kids

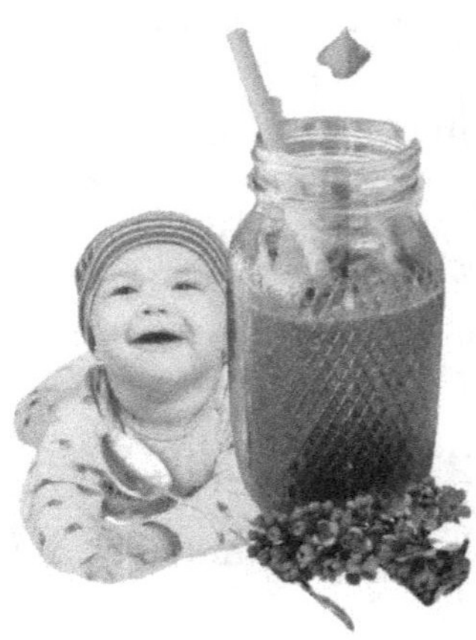

The Ultimate Guide to Break and Beat Sugar Cravings

Caroline Siebert

Copyright © 2023 Caroline Siebert

Table of Contents

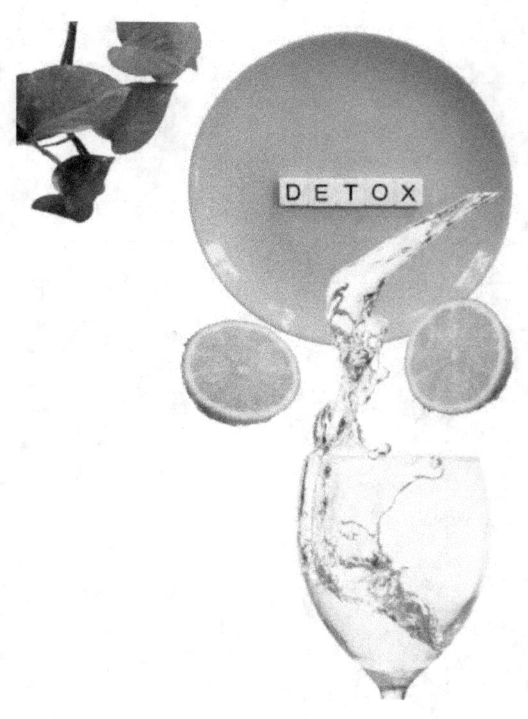
DETOX

INTRODUCTION

Six years ago, a family friend, Sarah, discovered that her 7-year-old daughter, Alexie, was becoming increasingly moody and had insomnia at night.

She also observed that her daughter was putting on weight and becoming less active. Out of concern for her daughter's health, Sarah took Alexie to the doctor, who found that she was showing early indicators of childhood obesity.

The news stunned and disturbed Sarah. Although she had always made an effort to provide Alexie with nutritious meals, she soon discovered that she had been giving her too much sugar.

She began looking at ways to assist Alexie in adopting healthier eating practices once she realized that something needed to change. This was happening at the time I started working on the concept of sugar detox.

A sugar detox entails avoiding all sugar-containing meals and beverages for a defined amount of time, often two to four weeks, in order to reset the body's desires and enhance general health.

When Sarah decided to give it a try, the results astounded her. Alexia's mood and behavior significantly improved after just a few days of the sugar detox. She was getting better nighttime sleep and was more energized during the day. She even began to love the nutritious foods she had previously avoided.

Sarah was pleased by the transformations she noticed in her kid and was aware that the sugar detox had an enormous impact on both her and her daughter.

Sarah now firmly believes in the benefits of a sugar detox for children. She encourages other parents to give it a try with their own kids so they can see the beneficial effect that it might have on their wellbeing and general health.

Just like Sarah, there are many parents out there who are struggling to get a perfect diet that will help their kids detox from sugar.

This is understandable because it can sometimes be so heartbreaking when you discover that what is causing a problem for your child is the sugar in his or her favorite beverages.

In this book, we will go over the fundamentals of a sugar detox for kids, including why it's crucial, early indications that your child needs one, and tips for an efficient detox.

This book will also provide you with some healthy sugar substitutes and urge you to start a sugar detox for your kid to ensure their health for the rest of their life.

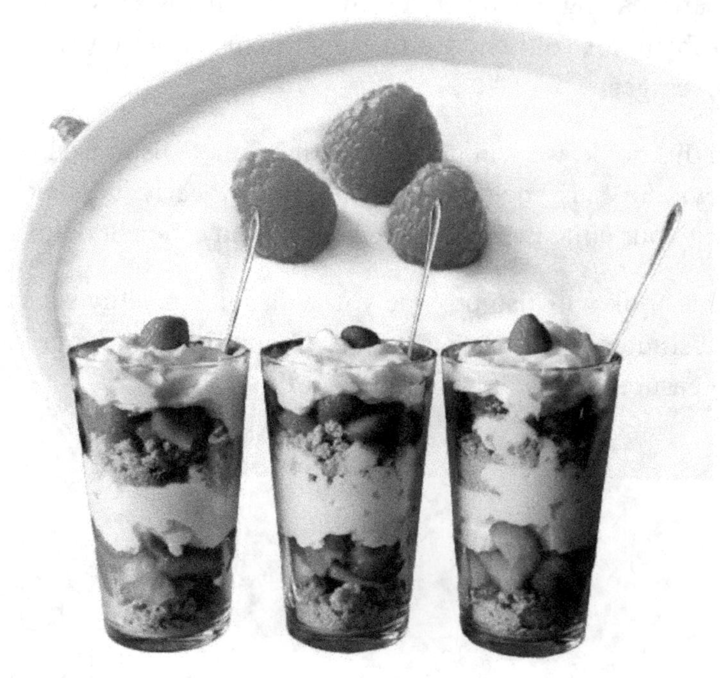

CHAPTER ONE

Understanding Sugar Detox

Sugar detox refers to the process of eliminating all sources of processed sugar from one's diet for an extended period of time.

This usually entails avoiding processed foods, sweets, and sugary drinks while replacing them with whole foods like fruits, vegetables, lean protein, and healthy fats.

A sugar detox is intended to reset the body's sugar cravings and improve overall health. When we consume a lot of sugar, our bodies get used to the constant influx of glucose and develop insulin resistance, which can lead to a variety of health issues like obesity, diabetes, and heart disease.

We can give our bodies a chance to reset and improve our overall wellness by reducing or eliminating added sugar from our diets. This can result in advantages such as an improved mood, better sleep, more energy, and better digestion.

Sugar detoxes can last anywhere from one week to several months, with some people opting for a one-week detox while others may choose to eliminate sugar from their diets for several months.

While a sugar detox can be a good way to get started on a healthier lifestyle, it is not a long-term solution. Once the detox is complete, it is necessary to continue eating healthy and limiting added or processed sugars as much as possible in order to maintain the detox's benefits.

Sugar detox can be difficult, particularly during the first few days as your body adjusts to the lack of sugar. Withdrawal symptoms such as headaches, fatigue, and irritability may arise in some people.

These symptoms, however, usually go away after a few days, and many people report feeling more energized and clear-headed after a sugar detox.

It's vital to recognize that not all sugars are created equal. While added sugars should be avoided to the greatest extent possible, natural sugars found in fruits and vegetables are an essential component of a healthy diet.

It is essential that you keep eating fruits and vegetables while on a sugar detox to ensure your body receives the nutrients it needs.

When removing sugar from your diet, it is also important to carefully read food labels. Many processed foods contain added sugars, even those marketed as "healthy." Ingredients such as high-fructose corn syrup, cane sugar, and maltodextrin should be avoided.

A sugar detox can aid in weight loss in addition to improving overall health. A high sugar intake can result in weight gain and difficulty losing weight. Many people find it easier to lose weight and keep it off when they eliminate added sugar.

It's important to note that sugar detox isn't for everyone, especially those with underlying health issues like diabetes. If you're thinking about doing a sugar detox, talk to your doctor first to make sure it's safe for you.

Generally speaking, a sugar detox can be an effective tool for establishing healthier eating habits and improving overall health.

While reducing or eliminating added sugars from your diet may be tough at first, the benefits are well worth the effort.

Why Your Kids Need Sugar Detox

Sugar detox is an active strategy for children to consider because excessive sugar consumption can have serious negative effects on their health.

Every day, the average American child consumes an alarming amount of sugar, frequently exceeding the recommended daily allowance. Excess sugar consumption has been linked to a number of health issues, including obesity, type 2 diabetes, and heart disease.

Sugar consumption is linked to weight gain and obesity, which is one of the main reasons why a sugar detox is important for kids. When we eat sugar, our bodies convert it into glucose, which is then used for energy or stored as fat.

Excess sugar consumption can result in a glucose overload in the body, which can lead to weight gain and obesity.

Childhood obesity rates in the United States have tripled since the 1970s, according to the Centers for Disease Control and Prevention (CDC), with one in every five children now classified as obese.

Obesity is a serious health concern because it can lead to a variety of health issues, such as type 2 diabetes, heart disease, and certain types of cancer.

Type 2 diabetes is a chronic disease in which the body develops resistance to insulin, a hormone that regulates blood sugar levels. Too much sugar intake can lead to insulin resistance, which can result to type 2 diabetes if proper care is not taken.

More than 34 million Americans have diabetes, according to the American Diabetes Association, with type 2 diabetes accounting for 90–95% of all cases.

Type 2 diabetes can result in serious health issues such as nerve damage, kidney damage, and vision problems.

High sugar intake can increase the risk of heart disease. Excess sugar consumption can result in high blood pressure, high cholesterol, and inflammation, which can all contribute to heart disease.

Heart disease is the leading cause of death in the United States, accounting for one in every four deaths each year, according to the American Heart Association.

Sugar detox is essential for kids because it can aid in the prevention of these serious health issues. Kids can reduce their risk of weight gain, type 2 diabetes, and heart disease by eliminating added sugars from their diets.

A sugar detox can also help improve mood, sleep, and energy levels, leading to improved academic performance and overall well-being.

CHAPTER TWO

Is sugar bad for your kids?

Sugar has been a contested issue in recent years, and for good reason. Every day, the average American child consumes an alarming amount of sugar, frequently exceeding the recommended daily allowance.

Excess sugar consumption can cause a variety of health problems, prompting many parents to wonder, "Is sugar bad for my kids?"

The short answer is that sugar can be harmful to your children. Let's look at why this is so.

We enjoy adding sugar to our juices, smoothies, and many of the foods we eat on a daily basis to give our taste buds a boost.

But the hidden sweet danger lurking behind these extras is enormous. Why? There are numerous reasons for this.

Here are four reasons why your child should avoid the sugar rush:

There is no nutritional value

Sugar has no nutritional value, so it is merely an empty calorie. However, when combined with other food products, sugar can significantly increase the number of calories in that food. Sugar is not a good source of energy because it has no nutritional value.

Weight gain

According to studies, even if you exercise regularly, a high sugar intake can lead to unhealthy weight gain. How? Sugar raises the calorie content of your food, resulting in weight gain.

Although it is a common misconception that sugar causes weight gain, Yes, it does not. Consuming too much sugar can result leptin resistance. Leptin, a hormone that regulates hunger and resistance, causes your body to eat more food than it should.

Tooth decay

According to studies, a high sugar intake can lead to unhealthy weight gain even if you exercise regularly. How? Sugar increases the calorie content of your food, which leads to weight gain.

Although it is a common misconception, sugar does not cause weight gain. Excess sugar intake can result in leptin resistance. Leptin, a hunger and resistance hormone, causes your body to eat more food than it should.

Diabetics

The fact that sugar causes diabetes is not a secret. Sugar causes insulin resistance, which in turn raises glucose levels in the body and leads to diabetes.

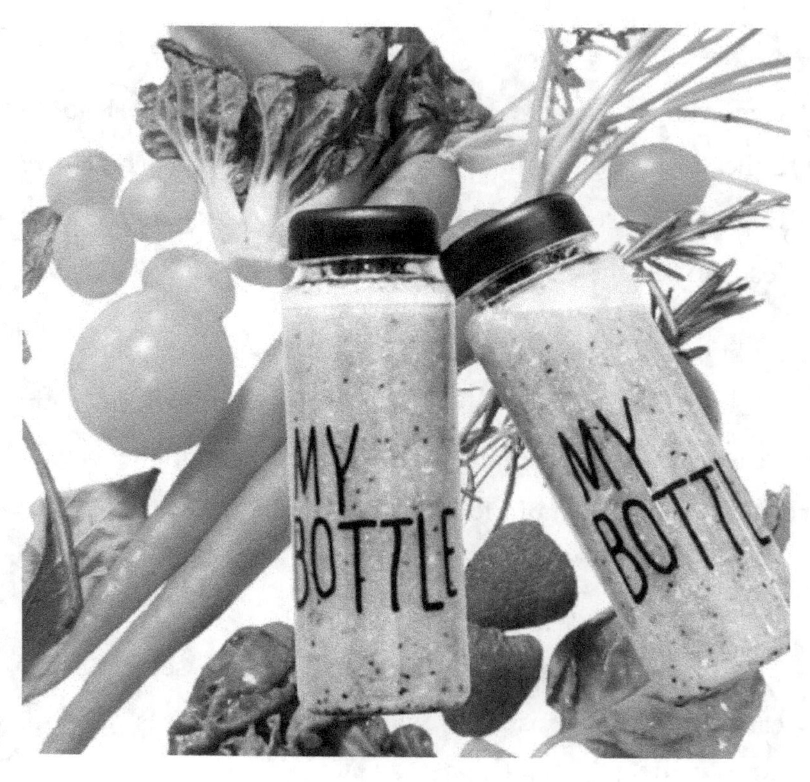
MY
BOTTLE
MY
BOTTL

CHAPTER THREE

Signs That Your Child Needs a Sugar Detox

There are several signs that your child may require a sugar detox:

Constant Cravings: If your child is constantly craving sugary foods and beverages, this could indicate that they are consuming too much sugar.

Energy Crash: If your child has a sudden drop in energy and appears tired or sluggish after consuming sugary foods or drinks, this could be a sign that they need a sugar detox.

Mood Swings: Excess sugar consumption in children can cause mood swings and irritability. If your child's mood appears to be affected by sugar consumption, it may be time for a sugar detox.

Dental Issues: If your child has frequent dental issues, such as cavities or gum disease, it could be a sign that their sugar intake is excessive.

Weight Gain: Excess sugar consumption in children can lead to weight gain and obesity. If your child is having trouble losing weight, it may be time to consider a sugar detox.

Poor Concentration: Excess sugar consumption can also impair your child's ability to concentrate and focus. If you notice your child struggling in school or having difficulty staying focused, it could be a sign that they need to reduce their sugar intake.

Skin Issues: Excess sugar consumption can result in skin issues such as acne, eczema, or rashes. If your child has these types of skin problems, it may be worth considering a sugar detox to see if it helps.

Digestive Issues: Excess sugar consumption can cause digestive issues such as bloating, gas, and constipation. If your child is exhibiting these symptoms, a sugar detox may be in order to help reset their digestive system.

Difficulty Sleeping: Too much sugar can also interfere with your child's sleep patterns. If your child is having trouble falling or staying asleep, a sugar detox may be worth considering to see if it improves their sleep quality.

You can help your child's overall health and wellbeing by recognizing these signs and taking steps to reduce their sugar intake.

A sugar detox can assist your child in developing healthier eating habits while also lowering their risk of developing health problems associated with excessive sugar consumption.

Behavioral Changes

Hyperactivity is a common behavioral change associated with excessive sugar consumption. A child who consumes too much sugar may become restless, fidgety, and unable to sit still. They may also struggle to pay attention and stay on task.

In addition to the behavioral changes mentioned earlier, excessive sugar consumption in children can lead to anxiety and depression.

Sugar can disrupt the balance of neurotransmitters in the brain, causing changes in mood and emotional regulation.

Furthermore, consuming an excessive amount of sugar on a regular basis can have long-term consequences for a child's behavior and mental health.

According to research, children who consume a lot of sugar are more likely to develop anxiety and depression symptoms later in life.

Addiction is another potential behavioral change associated with excessive sugar consumption. Sugar is highly addictive, and regular consumption can lead to cravings and withdrawal symptoms when it is not available.

When children are unable to access sugary foods and drinks, they may become irritable or upset, which can lead to a cycle of overconsumption and negative behavior.

You can help your child avoid these negative behavioral changes and promote better mental health and emotional regulation by reducing their sugar intake and promoting healthy eating habits.

Encouraging your child to eat a balanced diet rich in fruits, vegetables, and whole grains can help them develop a positive relationship with food and lower their risk of developing chronic health problems linked to excessive sugar consumption.

Another negative effect of too much sugar on a child's behavior is the possibility of decreased cognitive function. Sugar consumption has been linked to cognitive impairments such as poor memory, slower information processing, and a shorter attention span.

These cognitive changes have the potential to significantly impact a child's academic performance and overall learning ability.

Excessive sugar consumption in children can also lead to social and emotional problems. Children who consume a lot of sugar are more likely to have social issues, such as difficulty making friends or interacting with others.

This could be because of the effect sugar has on behavior and emotional regulation, as well as the possibility of addiction and cravings.

Lastly, excessive sugar consumption can harm a child's dental health. Sugary foods and beverages can cause tooth decay, which can result in pain, discomfort, and other dental issues. These problems can impair a child's ability to eat and speak comfortably, affecting their social and emotional well-being.

Physical Changes

Excessive sugar consumption can have a range of negative physical effects on a child's body. Here are some of the visible changes that can happen:

Poor nutrition: Consuming large amounts of sugar can displace other important nutrients in a child's diet, leading to poor nutrition. Children who consume too much sugar may not be getting enough vitamins, minerals, and other important nutrients that are essential for growth and development.

Fatigue: Consuming too much sugar can cause a spike in blood sugar levels, followed by a crash. This can lead to feelings of fatigue and low energy, which can affect a child's ability to perform daily activities.

Skin problems: Excessive sugar consumption can also lead to skin problems such as acne and premature aging. This is because sugar can cause inflammation in the body, which can contribute to these skin issues.

Increased risk of asthma: Studies have shown that children who consume a lot of sugar are more likely to develop asthma.

Hormonal imbalances: In children, a high sugar intake can lead to hormonal imbalances. This can have an impact on growth and development as well as other bodily functions.

Insulin resistance: Too much sugar in a child's diet can cause the body to become resistant to insulin, a hormone that helps regulate blood sugar levels. This can result in insulin resistance, which increases the risk of developing type 2 diabetes.

Increased inflammation: Eating a lot of sugar can cause inflammation in the body. This can lead to a variety of health issues, including heart disease, arthritis, and other chronic diseases.

Weakened immune system: Excess sugar consumption can also weaken the immune system, making it more difficult for a child's body to fight off infections and illnesses

Fatty liver disease development: A high sugar intake can cause fat to accumulate in the liver, leading to a condition known as fatty liver disease. This can harm the liver and increase the risk of developing liver disease later in life.

Increased risk of allergies and eczema: Studies have shown that children who consume a lot of sugar are more likely to develop allergies and eczema.

Growth retardation: A high-sugar diet can also impair a child's growth and development. Sugar consumption can lead to malnutrition by replacing nutrient-dense foods, resulting in poor growth and development.

Obesity: is one of the most well-known side effects of excessive sugar consumption. When a child consumes an excessive amount of sugar, the body stores the excess as fat.

This can lead to weight gain and obesity over time, increasing the risk of a variety of health issues such as heart disease, diabetes, and certain cancers.

Risk of heart disease: Excess sugar consumption has been linked to an increased risk of heart disease, even in children. Excess sugar consumption can result in high blood pressure, high cholesterol, and other heart disease risk factors.

Increased risk of certain cancers: Excess sugar consumption has also been linked to an increased risk of certain cancers, including liver, pancreatic, and colon cancer.

Excessive sugar consumption can also harm a child's bone health, increasing the risk of osteoporosis and other bone-related problems later in life.

Hormonal imbalances: Sugar can also disrupt a child's hormonal balance, resulting in issues such as early puberty and other reproductive issues.

Excessive sugar consumption can also increase the risk of non-alcoholic fatty liver disease, a condition that can lead to liver damage and other serious health problems.

Sugary foods and drinks frequently replace nutrient-dense foods like fruits, vegetables, and whole grains, so a high-sugar diet can lead to nutrient deficiencies.

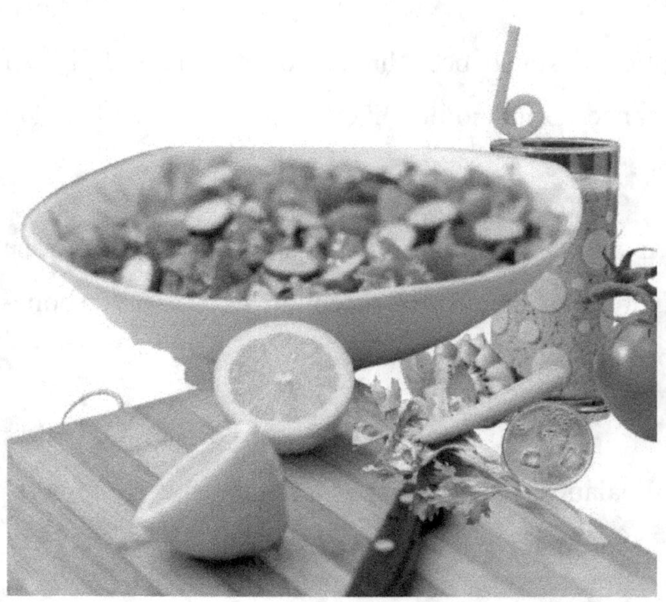

CHAPTER FOUR

Benefits of a Sugar Detox For Kids

Here are some advantages of a sugar detox for children:

1. Improved cognitive performance and mood

2. Improved sleep quality

3. Weight loss and a lower risk of obesity-related health problems

4. Reduced tooth decay and cavity risk

5. Improved overall physical health, including better immune function and a lower risk of chronic diseases

6. Improved concentration and behavior

7. Improved digestion and gut health

8. Increased intake of nutrient-dense foods for more consistent energy levels throughout the day.

9. Creating healthier eating habits for life

10. Reduced inflammation: A high-sugar diet can cause inflammation in the body, which can contribute to a variety of health issues. A sugar detox can aid in the reduction of inflammation and the promotion of overall health.

11. Improved liver function: The liver is in charge of the body's sugar processing and metabolization. When a child consumes an excessive amount of sugar, his or her liver may become overworked and damaged. Sugar detoxification can improve liver function and prevent liver disease.

12. Better mood and behavior: Excess sugar consumption in children can cause mood swings and behavioral issues. Parents can help their children have more stable moods and better behavior by reducing their sugar intake.

13. Enhanced athletic performance: A high-sugar diet can cause energy spikes and crashes, which can have a negative impact on athletic performance. A sugar detox can help balance out energy levels and improve athletic performance.

14. Improved mental health: Excess sugar consumption has been linked to an increased risk of depression, anxiety, and other mental health issues in children. Parents can help their children's mental health and well-being by limiting their sugar intake.

15. Improved skin health: Excess sugar consumption has been linked to skin problems such as acne and eczema. A sugar detox can improve skin health and lower the risk of these issues.

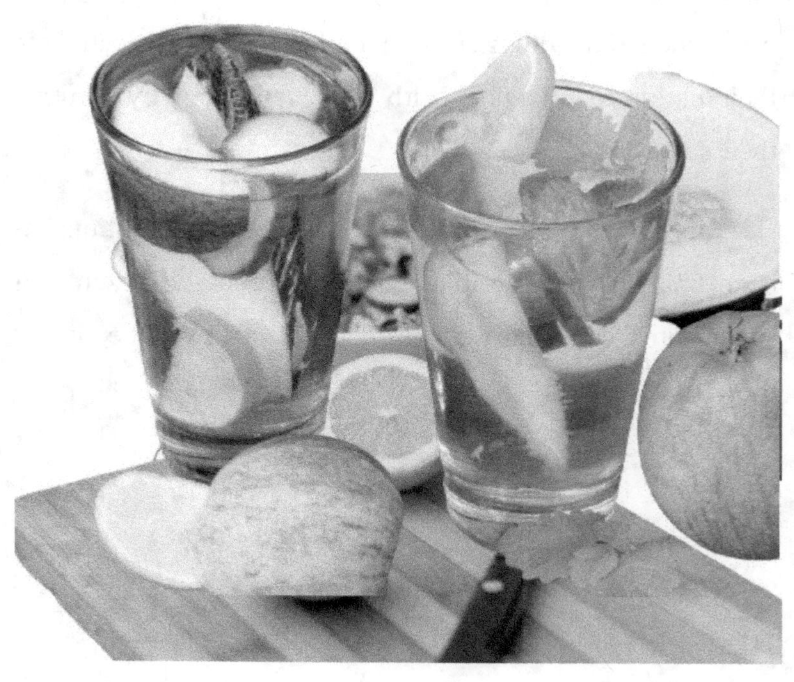

CHAPTER FIVE

Tips For Successful Sugar Detox For Kids

Here are some pointers for a successful sugar detox for kids:

Begin gradually: It can be challenging to go from a high-sugar diet to a sugar-free diet overnight. Begin by gradually reducing your child's sugar intake over several weeks or months.

Focus on whole foods: Instead of relying on sugary processed foods, focus on whole foods like fruits, vegetables, whole grains, and lean protein. These foods are naturally low in sugar and contain a variety of important nutrients.

Examine the labels carefully: Sugar can be found in a variety of foods, including those marketed as healthy or natural. Read labels carefully to identify hidden sugar sources and avoid foods with added sugars.

Limit or eliminate these beverages in favor of water, milk, or unsweetened alternatives: Sugary drinks, such as soda, fruit juice, and sports drinks, are among the most common sources of sugar in children's diets. It's important to limit or replace these beverages in their diets.

Involve your children in the sugar detox process by having them assist in meal planning, select healthy snacks, and prepare their own food. This can help them develop a stronger appreciation for healthy eating while also making the process more enjoyable and engaging.

Keep healthy snacks on hand, such as fresh fruit, vegetables, and nuts, for when your child needs a quick and healthy snack. This can help keep them away from sugary snacks and treats.

Celebrate your child's accomplishments in lowering their sugar intake and making healthier food choices. This can help reinforce positive behaviors and motivate them to make healthier choices in the future.

: It is critical to set attainable goals for your child's sugar detox. Setting unrealistic expectations can make it difficult for your child to meet them, leading to feelings of frustration or failure. Set little, achievable goals that you can develop on over time.

: A sugar detox can be more successful if the entire family participates. Make it a family effort to cut back on sugar and adopt healthier eating habits. This can provide support and accountability for your child while also benefiting the overall health of the family.

: Teach your child about the negative health effects of excess sugar, such as an increased risk of obesity, type 2 diabetes, and other chronic diseases. This can inspire them to make healthier choices and take charge of their health.

: Rewarding your child with sugar reinforces the idea that sugary treats are a desirable reward, making it more difficult for your child to break the cycle of sugar addiction. Instead, look for non-food rewards like extra playtime, a favorite activity, or a special outing.

Be a positive role model: Because children learn by example, it's critical for parents and caregivers to set a good example for healthy eating habits.

Model healthy behaviors such as eating a balanced diet, drinking water or milk instead of sugary drinks, and participating in family physical activity.

Parents and caregivers can help their children successfully complete a sugar detox and develop healthier eating habits that will benefit them for the rest of their lives by following these tips.

CHAPTER SIX

Healthy Alternatives to Sugar

Finding healthy alternatives to sugar can help kids reduce their sugar intake. Here are some safer substitutes to sugar:

Fresh fruit is naturally sweet and contains important vitamins and minerals that are necessary for growing bodies. Encourage your child to eat fresh fruit instead of sugary treats as a snack or dessert.

Yogurt with honey: Plain yogurt is high in protein and calcium, but it can be too sour for some children. To sweeten it up without adding too much sugar, drizzle it with honey.

Homemade popsicles: Instead of buying sugary store-bought popsicles, make your own at home with fresh fruit and yogurt or coconut milk. Freeze in popsicle molds for a healthy treat.

Dark chocolate contains less sugar than milk chocolate and also contains antioxidants that are beneficial to one's health. For maximum health benefits, choose dark chocolate with a high percentage of cocoa solids.

Whole grain crackers with nut butter: For a high-protein, fiber-rich snack, try whole grain crackers with nut butter like almond or peanut butter. The nut butter's healthy fats can help children feel full and satisfied.

Smoothies: Smoothies are an excellent way to consume fruits and vegetables while still enjoying a sweet treat. Blend a variety of fruits and vegetables with yogurt or milk for a nutritious and tasty snack or meal replacement.

Water flavored with fruit or herbs: Instead of sugary drinks, encourage your child to drink water flavored with fruit slices or herbs like mint or basil. This can provide a refreshing flavor without adding additional sugar.

Homemade granola bars: Many store-bought granola bars contain a lot of sugar. Make your own at home with natural sweeteners like honey or maple syrup, and add ingredients like nuts, seeds, and dried fruit for extra nutrition.

Baked apples or pears: For a warm and comforting dessert, bake apples or pears with cinnamon and honey drizzle. This can provide natural sweetness without the use of excessive sugar.

Instead of potato chips or other processed snacks, try making your own chips out of fruits and vegetables. Simply thinly slice them, toss with olive oil and sea salt, and bake for a crispy and nutritious snack.

Coconut water is a natural source of electrolytes and can be a great substitute for sugary sports drinks. It hydrates without adding sugar, making it a healthier option for active kids.

Chia pudding: Chia seeds are high in fiber and protein, and when soaked in liquid, they take on the consistency of pudding. Make chia pudding with coconut milk or almond milk and natural sweeteners like honey or maple syrup.

Date Paste: Dates are a natural sweetener that can be blended into a paste and used in recipes like cookies and muffins in place of sugar. They are high in fiber and vitamin content.

Nut butters like almond or peanut butter, for example, can add natural sweetness and protein to snacks like apple slices or rice cakes.

Coconut cream: Without the added sugars found in traditional versions, coconut cream can be used as a natural sweetener in recipes such as frosting or whipped cream.

Herbal teas: such as chamomile or peppermint, can satisfy a sweet craving without containing the added sugars found in flavored teas or sugary drinks.

Unsweetened applesauce: can be used in place of sugar in recipes such as muffins and pancakes, and it adds natural sweetness and moisture.

Cinnamon: Cinnamon can add natural sweetness to foods like oatmeal or yogurt without adding sugar. This is also helpful when it comes to blood sugar control

Honey: Honey is a natural sweetener that can be used sparingly to flavor foods like oatmeal or toast. It also contains antibacterial and antioxidant properties.

Pure maple syrup: This is a natural sweetener high in antioxidants and minerals like zinc and manganese. It can be used sparingly to sweeten foods like pancakes or yogurt.

Stevia: This is a natural sweetener derived from the leaves of the stevia plant that can be used in recipes in place of sugar or added to drinks. There are no calories in it, and it has no effect on blood sugar levels.

Dates: Dates are a natural sweetener that can be added to smoothies or baked with. They also have a high fiber, potassium, and antioxidant content.

Coconut sugar: Coconut sugar is a natural sweetener that has a lower glycemic index than regular sugar, which means it won't cause blood sugar spikes. It can be baked with or added to coffee or tea.

Molasses: A byproduct of sugar production, molasses contains vitamins and minerals like iron, calcium, and potassium. It can be used in baking or as a natural sweetener in oatmeal or yogurt.

It's important to remember that even these natural sweeteners should be used in moderation, and that the goal of a sugar detox is to reduce overall intake of added sugars.

By incorporating a variety of healthy alternatives to sugar into your child's diet, you can help them develop a taste for natural sweetness and establish healthy habits that will benefit their overall health and well-being.

Encouragement To Start A Sugar Detox For Your Child

It can be difficult to encourage your child to begin a sugar detox, but as a parent, you must prioritize your child's health and well-being. Here are some suggestions to help you persuade your child to begin a sugar detox:

If you're thinking about starting a sugar detox for your child, make sure you approach the topic positively and supportively.

Instead of making your child feel guilty or ashamed about their current eating habits, focus on the advantages of making healthier choices.

Encourage your child to participate in the process by including them in meal planning and grocery shopping so they can learn more about the foods they consume.

Remember that a sugar detox does not have to be all or nothing. Small changes can make a big difference, and even reducing your child's sugar intake slightly can improve their health.

You can help your child develop healthy eating habits that will benefit them for the rest of their lives if you have patience, persistence, and a positive attitude.

Encourage your child to begin a sugar detox by educating them on the effects of sugar on their health. Because children may not fully comprehend the long-term consequences of a high-sugar diet, it is critical to explain to them how sugar can lead to obesity, type 2 diabetes, and heart disease.

By involving your child in grocery shopping and meal preparation, you can also help them develop a greater appreciation for healthy, nutritious foods.

Encourage them to eat fruits, vegetables, and whole grains, and allow them to assist you in preparing meals and snacks. This can make them feel more invested in the process and more willing to experiment with new, healthy foods.

Making a sugar detox a fun and exciting challenge is another way to encourage your child to start one. You can make a chart or a tracking system to help your child keep track of their progress and reward them for reaching certain milestones.

You can also involve their classmates or friends in a friendly competition to see who can make the healthiest choices.

When encouraging your child to begin a sugar detox, the most important thing is to approach it with a positive and supportive attitude.

Make it clear to your child that you are there to support and encourage them and that you are proud of them for pursuing a healthier lifestyle.

You can assist your child in making the transition to a healthier, happier life with patience, persistencse, and a positive attitude.

Furthermore, as a parent, it is critical to set a good example by making healthy choices and limiting your own sugar intake. Children often mimic their parents' behavior, so if they see you making positive changes, they may be more willing to follow suit.

You can also involve your child's healthcare provider in the process and seek advice and support from them.

Your child's doctor can provide additional guidance on the specific dietary changes that would be most beneficial for your child's individual needs, as well as monitor and encourage them along the way.

Remember that transitioning to a healthier diet can be a slow process that requires patience and consistency. It may take some time for your child to adjust to new tastes and textures, but with patience and positivity, you can help them develop lifelong healthy habits.

It's vital to recognize and celebrate small victories along the way. Every step toward a healthier lifestyle is a positive step, and by recognizing and celebrating these accomplishments, you can help your child stay motivated and encouraged to continue making good choices.

You can also make the sugar detox process enjoyable for your child by involving them in meal planning and preparation. This can make them feel more empowered and invested in the process, as well as teach them valuable skills for making healthy choices on their own in the future.

Consider incorporating fruits and vegetables, whole grains, lean proteins, and healthy fats into your child's diet. To keep things interesting and exciting, experiment with new recipes and flavors.

Finally, keep in mind that a sugar detox is not about deprivation or strict rules. It is about making positive changes to improve your child's health and well-being, and it is critical to approach the process with kindness, compassion, and an emphasis on progress rather than perfection.

You can help your child develop a healthy relationship with food and set them on a path to lifelong wellness by doing so.

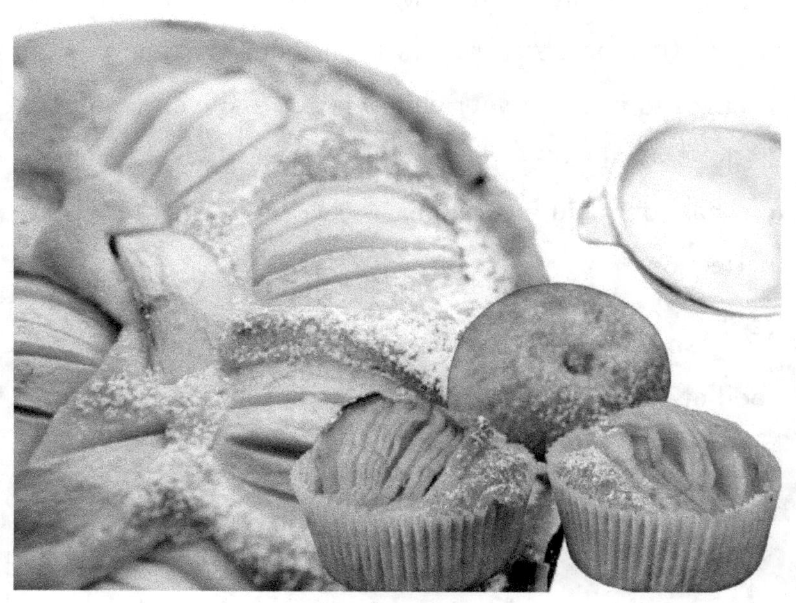

CHAPTER SEVEN

A 7-Day Sugar Detox Meal Plan For Kids

Sugar reduction in a child's diet is an important step toward a healthier lifestyle. A sugar detox meal plan can assist in replacing processed foods, sugary drinks, and snacks with wholesome, nutrient-dense meals.

This 7-day sugar detox meal plan for kids is intended to be simple to follow and delicious while also providing a well-balanced nutritional intake.

Tips for preparation:

It's critical to plan ahead of time before beginning the sugar detox meal plan. Here are some pointers:

Remove all sugary snacks, processed foods, and sugary drinks from your pantry and refrigerator.

Stock up on whole foods such as fresh fruits and vegetables, whole grains, lean protein sources, and healthy fats.

Plan your meals and snacks for the coming week, and prepare any ingredients ahead of time to save time.

Get your child involved in meal planning and preparation to teach them about healthy eating and foster an interest in cooking.

7-Day Sugar Detox Meal Plan for Kids:

Day 1:

Breakfast: Oatmeal with freshly prepared berries and almond milk

Snack: Apple slices with almond butter

Lunch: Turkey and creamy avocado wrap with whole-grain tortilla

Snack: Carrot sticks with hummus

Dinner: Salmon baked in the oven with roasted sweet potatoes and broccoli

Day 2:

Breakfast: Greek yogurt with sliced peaches and granola

Snack: Banana and walnuts

Lunch: Stir-fry chicken and vegetables with brown rice

Snack: Bell pepper strips with guacamole

Dinner: Turkey chili with mixed greens salad

Day 3:

Breakfast: Scrambled eggs with fresh spinach and whole-grain toast

Snack: Orange slices

Lunch: Tuna salad with whole-grain crackers

Snack: Celery sticks with almond butter

Dinner: Grilled chicken with oven-roasted carrots and quinoa

Day 4:

Breakfast: Smoothie bowl with freshly mixed berries, almond milk, and granola

Snack: Pear and cashews

Lunch: Egg salad with mixed greens on whole-grain bread

Snack: Cucumber slices with tzatziki dip

Dinner: Beef and vegetable stew with mixed greens salad

Day 5:

Breakfast: Cottage cheese with sliced peaches and whole-grain toast

Snack: Pineapple chunks

Lunch: Lentil soup with whole-grain crackers

Snack: Cherry tomatoes with mozzarella cheese

Dinner: Roasted chicken with roasted sweet potato and green beans

Day 6:

Breakfast: Veggie omelette with whole-grain toast

Snack: Grapefruit and pistachios

Lunch: Turkey and cheese roll-ups served with mixed greens

Snack: Sugar snap peas with hummus

Dinner: Whole grilled fish with oven-roasted asparagus and quinoa

Day 7:

Breakfast: Peanut butter and banana smoothie with chia seeds

Snack: Apple slices with cinnamon

Lunch: Black bean and vegetable salad with avocado dressing

Snack: Sliced cucumber with tzatziki dip

Dinner: Baked turkey meatballs served with garlic parmesan zucchini noodles and marinara sauce

CONCLUSION

A sugar detox can be a transformative experience for both you and your child. You can help improve their overall health and wellbeing, lower their risk of developing chronic illnesses, and set them on a path to lifelong wellness by reducing or eliminating sugar from their diet.

Throughout this book, we've discussed the numerous advantages of a sugar detox for kids, as well as the risks and dangers of excessive sugar consumption. We've talked about the signs that your child might need a sugar detox as well as tips and strategies for making the process go smoothly.

We've also looked into sugar alternatives like whole foods, natural sweeteners, and other tasty treats that can help satisfy your child's sweet tooth without compromising their health.

You can help your child make positive changes to their diet and lifestyle by following the advice and guidance in this book and putting them on a path to lifelong health and wellness. Remember to approach the process with patience, persistence, and optimism, and to celebrate your accomplishments along the way.

It's important to remember that a sugar detox is only the beginning of your child's healthy lifestyle. Encouraging them to make healthy choices for the rest of their lives will help them stay healthy and avoid chronic illnesses.

You can also keep your child involved in the process by allowing them to assist in the planning and preparation of healthy meals and snacks, as well as encouraging them to try new foods and flavors. This can help them develop a love of healthy, nutritious foods while also teaching them important skills for making their own healthy choices.

Finally, keep in mind that a sugar detox is not a one-size-fits-all solution. Every kid is unique, and what is suitable for one might not be suitable for another.

Be patient and flexible in your approach, and be willing to adjust your strategies as needed to meet the unique needs of your child.

Thank you for reading this book, and we wish you and your child the best of luck on your journey to a healthier, happier life.